HOW TO

BUILD MUSCLE

WITHOUT

WEIGHTS IN 21

DAYS

HOW TO BUILD MUSCLE WITHOUT WEIGHTS

Hey Pamela why would anyone want to workout without weights? Everyone knows that using weights and machines is the fastest most efficient way to gain size and strength. While this is true, there are many reasons why someone would want to, or even be forced to train for a while without the benefit of using weights. Someone working long hours trying to support his family may not have the time to get to a commercial gym, and may not have the extra space or money to set up a good home gym. Also, someone who has to travel quite often for business might prefer getting a good workout in his or her hotel room rather then wandering the streets of America asking "Where's a gym?".

Let's face it there are times (vacations, etc.) when all of us can't easily get to a gym. There are also many trainees (beginners or athletes training for boxing, baseball or some other sport) who aren't trying to get a lot of muscular bulk but want the type of strength, endurance and definition that calisthenic exercise offers. These exercises can also be preformed anytime, anywhere and you can do them over your entire life to keep fit. The idea behind this course is - If for some reason you do workout without weights, what is the most efficient and result producing way to do it? You can use these exercises in many ways: To build muscle, to maintain muscle you already have, in combination with your weight training to add variety and a change of pace, as a warm-up or pump-up routine, to ease back into training after a layoff or injury, etc., etc.

"The original reason was to help out one of my best friends at the time, who also happened to be the person that inspired me to start training by seeing the great progress he was making. Let's call him Dave, mostly because that was his name, I believe he prefers to be called David these days but back then he was still good old Joe.

Anyway, one day Dave's father forbid him to workout with weights anymore, he gave Dave some reasons for this decision but I think the real reason was that he didn't like the idea that his 13 year old son was getting a little too big and strong to be easily controlled and he better do something about it before he gets any bigger. The funny part was that his father didn't object to him doing push-ups or other freehand exercises, only weight training was forbidden, I'm sure he figured that at best Joe would be able to maintain the muscle he had but he wouldn't get any bigger. Joe was very distraught by the situation, convinced that his muscles were doomed to waste away to nothing, but I was sure there was some way to make those exercise more intense and maybe he could even gain some size. I came up with some ideas and tried to tell Dave about them but he didn't seem too interested, his attitude was like "Hey, I know more about training then this guy, I'm the one who got him started. And besides I don't have time to listen to this I'm too busy feeling sorry for myself and performing satanic rituals to curse my dad-''.

Dave never used my ideas but I did many times over the years, whenever I used calisthenics, and always got good results. I got even more ideas, a few years back, after reading the famous "Dynamic-Tension Course" by Charles Atlas. I found an old comic book and decided to write to the address and see if the course was still available, much to my delight it was and I ordered it. I ordered it mostly as a collectors piece and novelty item, like owning a part of American pop culture. Who could forget those great advertisements like, "The insult that made a man out of 'Mac'.", "Who else wants a He-Man body?" or "In just 7 days, I can make you a Man.", I was also curious as to what was this Dynamic-Tension method exactly. I have always believed that - Only a fool thinks he knows everything and that a wise man never stops learning., so there was a possibility that I could find some good information in this "old, outdated course". I read the course and found it quite interesting, I was slightly disappointed to find out that Dynamic-Tension is really just some calisthenics and some isometric exercises. And while I'm sure they would do a lot for 198 lb weaklings", what can they do for someone who's already fairly big and strong? This got me thinking again about the same thing, how can these exercises be made more intense. Since then I came up with a few more ideas and now it's time to end the history lesson and share them with you."

This is a story as shared by one of my acquaintance, after which I have taken much efforts to carry out the proficiency of his talk

THE TECHNIQUES

(1) The first technique is to just do the exercises in the traditional manner, I know you can do 60, 80 even 100 reps but that's the idea, grind out as many reps as you can this will build up your

endurance and give your muscles a change of pace. And while this most likely won't give you any extra size right away, when you go back to weight training with heavy weights and lower reps you may be sup prised that you are now gaining faster then before. A few years ago some top bodybuilders were talking about a technique they called "100's", they reduced the weight and did literally 100 reps on all their exercises, they claimed it brought about certain physiological changes that made the muscles more responsive to later heavier training. It's worth a try, especially if you're going to be doing calisthenics anyway.

(2) Another way to get more results from these exercises is, right after a set flex hard the muscles just worked, flex as hard as you can and hold for at least a count of 10. Arnold talked extensively about "Posing as exercise" and the use of "Iso-Tension"(Iso means - Equal; the same, and Tension means - To tighten; stiffen; contract. So Iso-Tension is simply contacting the muscles and holding in the same place - no movement.) he said that it really

gives the body a more chiseled look, reaches areas that training misses and will make muscular contractions while training more intense, and more isolated. All good reasons to try this technique.

A better variation of this is to flex the muscles you are working first, get them good and tired and then do the exercise, thus Pre-Fatiguing them. For example flex the chest or triceps muscles as hard as you can, then immediately do a set of push-ups. Feels different doesn't it? It's a lot harder and produces much better results.

(3) Another technique is to reduce the rest time between exercises, let's say you start with 60 seconds after a while cut it down to 45 then 30, then 15, etc. How about no rest between sets, a whole cycle of calisthenics all done nonstop that makes it way more intense.

Also try it this way - do one set, let's say of chin-ups, go until the muscles are really tired or even to total failure wait only a few seconds and then do another set. How many reps did you do on your second set? Only 4 or 5 I bet, that's about what you'd do if you were doing some heavy pull-downs. You should see some growth from this style. Make it even more intense by increasing the reps on the first set and by decreasing the rest time before the second set, this is using the Rest-Pause method without weights.

(4) Why not simply add some weight, just because it's not metal disks doesn't matter your body can't tell the difference. Put some heavy books on your back and do push-ups, or even your 8 year old son, he likes to play

horsy. Get your wife or girlfriend (but not both at the same time, that could be trouble) to sit on your shoulders while you do squats. Do donkey calf raises, get creative there's always a way to add some more resistance.

(5) How about using only one limb at a time, like doing one legged squats, one arm chin-ups, one arm push-ups, etc.. It takes some balance but it definitely makes it harder and puts on more muscle.

(6) Slow-Motion training is becoming popular again, try taking a full 12 seconds for the positive phase and 6

seconds for the negative phase of each rep. Don't lock out in the top position and don't rest in the bottom position, change smoothly from the positive to the negative. This is using Slow Continuous Tension, how many chin-up can you do this way? Not many I bet, it's intense.

(7) This last technique is based on what I thought Dynamic-Tension was before I read the course, Dynamic means - Dealing with motion, and we know from before that Tension is simply contraction. Therefore true Dynamic- Tension would be flexing the

muscles hard while also moving, martial artists use a form of this to increase punching power.

Let's try to use this applied to our freehand workout, do your push-ups nice and slow while flexing hard your pectorals, shoulders, triceps, biceps and even your lats and forearms. When doing chin-ups flex hard your lats, shoulders, biceps, triceps and even chest and forearms. Do deep knee bends and flex hard your quadriceps, hamstrings, glutes, hips and even calves. Keep the tension hard and steady, it will take some practice to do it all together, but the incredible pump and muscle growth you will get from it will be well worth your while. Increase reps and sets; decrease rest time. The more you do an exercise, the more you'll increase the metabolic stress you put on your muscles. Do more reps and sets of bodyweight exercises than you'd typically do at the gym with weights for similar results. You also want to limit breaks between those reps and sets, too, without sacrificing proper form. This puts more stress on the muscle, promoting growth. In fact, research shows that low-load resistance training (with a light weight or bodyweight) combined with little rest may enhance metabolic stress and increase muscle size even more than lifting heavy weights and taking longer breaks. If you typically lift weights for about eight reps in the gym, try doing that same move for 20 reps at home with just your body.

(8). Change the angle or tempo of the exercise. To increase microtrauma, try taking your lunges for a walk or stepping out on a diagonal. Or add an incline or decline to your push-ups, suggests Galbraith. Changing the angle can both incorporate other muscles into the move, but also work different parts of the same muscle group. It's also a good idea to slow down the eccentric or downward phase of an exercise (like when you lower to the bottom of a deadlift) and then explode up (quickly moving up from a deadlift or hinged position). Another option: Slow down the entire exercise. For example, lower into a squat on a count of three, holding at the bottom for three, then stand up on another count of three. This increases the time your muscle is under tension, meaning you're more likely to create microtraumas within your slow-twitch muscle fibers, which have more endurance capacity than fast-twitch fibers

(9). Add some holds and half-reps. This can add more metabolic stress to the muscles, thus resulting in more gains. For example, if lunges feel easy, hold the bottom of the movement (both knees bent 90 degrees) for a few seconds before standing up. Or, step back into your lunge, lift halfway up, then drop back down before you come back up to standing. Also, try stopping short of standing all the way up from a squat or lunge, or stop short of lowering all the way down in a glute bridge. This works because you're putting the muscle under tension for a longer period of time, or eliminating any points in the movement where the working muscle gets a break. Do more plyometrics. To increase the tension on your muscles, add some explosiveness to your moves. Squat jumps, lunge jumps, hinge jumps, burpees—they all count toward more muscle building. When a muscle is stretched, it leads to nerve firing that signals a concentric contraction (shortening of the muscle).

A quicker stretch (like what happens during the explosive portion of a plyometric exercise) leads to a stronger nerve firing and greater resulting contraction of the muscle. That stronger contraction means your muscle is working harder, and will likely result in more microtrauma and thus more gains. One study on young soccer players found that those who performed plyometric moves had similar muscle gains to those who did resistance training.

(10). Perform single-sided exercises. Switch your typical bilateral (or two-sided) exercises to unilateral (or one-sided) movements. That means turning a squat to a pistol squat, making your glute bridge a single-leg bridge, or turning your plank into a single arm (and/or leg) plank. These simple switches can increase the microtrauma to a muscle, as well as add more tension or load to that muscle, says Galbraith. Think about it: One side is handling all the weight rather than splitting it.

(11). Slow It Down In order to build muscle, you need to place enough stress on the muscles in order to break them down. Then as your rest and your muscles recover, you muscles will rebuild and become bigger and stronger. So in order to allow bodyweight exercises to place enough stress on your muscles, you need to make them as hard as possible. By making each rep really slow you will be placing maximum stress on the muscles. Perform each half of the rep for at least 10-12 seconds. Every now and again mix it up with an ultra-long rep of 20 seconds up, and 20 seconds down.

(12). Go To Failure Bodyweight exercises are a great way to shock your body into muscle growth, this is especially the case if you go to failure. Failure is the stage at which you cannot do another rep. So in addition to doing low number of reps slowly, try to do as many reps as possible. This is a great way to shock your body into muscle growth. Because after your muscles have recovered from these high reps, their endurance and strength will have improved and thus they will be able to handle more stress within your daily workouts.

(13). Flex The Muscle Before you perform a bodyweight exercise, try tiring out the muscles in advance by flexing them. Contract the muscles that you are about to be working for at least 30 seconds. Then when you are performing the exercises, pause at the moment of maximum muscle contraction to flex the muscles for a few more seconds. This flexing places extra stress on the muscles and makes them work harder, thus encouraging increased strength and muscle growth.

SOME SUGGESTED EXERCISES

Deep Knee Bends - Builds thighs, glutes, hips and great for lung power and endurance. With your feet about shoulder width apart, grab on to the edge of a sink (or something that will give you support) and while looking up slowly bend your knees and lower until your butt is just about touching the floor. Slowly stand up again using only your legs to lift you, keep your heals on the floor and do as many as you can. For variation you can place your feet wider or closer together, or do them one leg at a time.

Calf Raises - Do them on steps, put your toes on the edge of a step and hold on to the hand rail for balance, lower your heals to get a good stretch, then raise up on your toes as high as you can, lower and repeat for as many as you can. For variation try them in the squatted down position, one leg of a time or donkey style.

Chin-ups or Pull-ups - For building back, shoulders, and biceps. Grab a bar with an under hand grip and hang down getting a good stretcth in the lats, Pull up until your chest hits the bars, lower and repeat for as many. These can be easily be done in a park, school yard or on a doorway chin bar. Also try with an overhand grip, with one arm at a time, or even on monkey bars using a parallel grip (palms facing each other). For building chest, shoulders and triceps. Lie face down on the floor hands about shoulder width apart keep your palms turned inward slightly, push-up until your arms are straight, lower and repeat for reps. To make it more difficult elevate your feet. Also, try different hand placements (closer together or farther apart). They can also be done between chairs, this was the favorite exercise of Charles Atlas. Another variation is Dips between parallel bars.

Handstand Push-Ups - Great for shoulders and arms. Get into a handstand next to a wall, put your toes against the wall for balance, lower yourself until the top of your head touches the ground, push back up and repeat for many reps. Try both close and wide hand Placements.

Crunches - For firming abdominal and reducing stomach. Lie on your back with your legs bent and your heals close to your butt, put your chin on your chest and your hands behind your head. Raise your head up crunching your abs hard (you should only go about 1/3 of the way as compared to traditional sit-ups) lower and repeat for lots of reps.

Hyper -Extentions - For strengthening your lower back. Place a chair near a bed, while lying face down with your hips on the chair and your lower legs shoved between the mattress and box spring, put your hands behind your head and bend forward at the waist as far as you can, raise back up until your back is straight and repeat for reps.

Grip Exercise - To build forearms and hand strength. Use a store bought pocket hand gripper, or a hard rubber ball that fits in your hand, squeeze as hard as you can, relax and repeat for many reps. Also try just the thumb and one finger at a time, exercise each finger this way.

Push-ups. This is the second time Push upis coming up, andthas because of the relevance and effectivenss of push ups. If you want to learn how to build muscle without weights fast, then you should learn how to do the push-ups. At least 3 sets or 15 repetitions of push-ups can already help you develop your muscles particularly on your shoulders, chest and arms. Standing

Calf Raises This can be very helpful in strengthening and developing the proper shape of your legs. You may simply use a platform or even the staircases at your home in order to perform this exercise.

Bicycle Crunches If you wish to learn how to build muscle without weights fast as well as developing the muscles in the abdominal portion of your body, then this exercise should be included in your routine. Bicycle crunches can work on your upper and lower abdomen as well as your obliques. On your routines, make sure to do at least 3 sets with 15 repetitions for each leg to maintain the balance between each leg.

Squats This exercise is very helpful when trying to develop the muscles in the thighs as well as the legs. You may do this exercises for 3 sets with 15 repetitions each during your routine.

Calf Raises This exercise is very simple but it can help you improve the muscles on your calves. You may repeat this exercise up to 12 to 15 times every time you are doing your routines.

Lunges This is another thigh and leg exercise. This can also be done at least 12 to 15 times when doing your routines and you may also do it alternately.

Leg Raises This is an exercise which is good for the lower abs. Start off with 15 repetitions until you get used to it before gradually raising the number of repeats.

Cardiovascular exercises This should definitely be included in your exercise routine. If you really want to learn how to develop muscle without weights fast, then you should include this in your exercise as this can be very helpful. Make sure to spend several minutes swimming or running or doing any other cardiovascular exercises in order to increase your body's overall health and fitness.

Isometrics - Serious Muscle Training Without Weights

Isometrics - super fast way to increase muscle size & strength without using weights. Isometrics is perhaps the most under utilized and under rated method of exercise. It is perhaps the best method of strength training to be used in rehabilitation and can produce increases in strength and size where traditional, weight bearing, exercise regimes have failed. Isometric contraction, normally just called

ISOMETRICS, is one in which the muscle is activated, but instead of being allowed to lengthen or shorten, it is held at a constant length. This isometrics muscle contraction is not done through a range of movements but in a static position. Isometrics is based on the principles of creating muscular tension while opposing the force of an immovable object or gravity. Isometrics are done with high levels of intensity (70-100%) rather than repetitious movements typically for a period of 7-12 seconds. Once the muscle is relaxed after the contraction increases blood flow to the muscles occurs which equals more nutrition and energy uptake which in turn increases the muscle mass (size). Isometric exercise is a form of resistance training in which the participant uses the muscles of the body to exert a force either against an immovable object or to hold the muscle in a fixed position for a set duration of time. In this type of exercise, the muscle is contracted but does not change length during the exertion of force. Additionally the joint most closely associated with the effort remains static throughout the exercise. Isometric training has been around for centuries in such things as yoga and Chinese martial arts. Even Pilates utilizes isometric exercise as part of its training protocol. Isometrics is probably one of the very few exercise techniques that has been scientifically validated. At the Max Plank Institute in the 1950's Dr. Hettinger and Dr. Mueller conducted scientific research into the field of isometrics. Their study showed conclusively that isometrics can increase strength by as much as 300% in less than 30 days! Isometric

Workouts were originally made famous by Charles Atlas - although he branded it as "Dynamic Tension" and in recent years isometric workouts have made a huge comeback especially in the field of rehabilitation therapy. Several devices that use isometrics as the basis of the exercise protocol have been developed by Gert F Koebel including the Bullworker. Isometric contraction refers to the case of strength training, in which the muscles contract, but do not change their length. The name isometric comes from the words 'iso' meaning equal and 'metric' meaning distance. In contrary to other dynamic muscle contractions that involve change in position, isometric contraction is performed in a static position. Physical activities based on isometric muscle contraction are known isometric exercises. Sometimes weight lifters and professional bodybuilders will incorporate some isometrics into their workouts, often in order to break through barriers and to attain new levels of muscle strength which in turn leads to new and increased muscle mass.

Advantages of Isometric Contraction

Exercises Isometric exercises can be carried out virtually anywhere! You can do them whilst sitting watching TV, while sunbathing, while you wait in a traffic jam and well the list goes on and on. Everyday, we could if we want indulge in performing isometric contractions as a part of our day-to-day activities, such as carrying a suitcase or a carrier bag full of groceries. Isometrics are particularly beneficial with those with back pain as the muscles can be developed without further damaging the back and the resultant gains in (say) abdominal strength help to alleviate the stress on your back which in turn helps the back to heal as your stronger abs take the strain away from your injured back. Often the main advantages are seen as maximal muscular contraction in a short space of time. I use isometric training with many of my corporate clients who simply do not have the time to go to the gym.Isometric contraction exercises lasting for 7 - 10 seconds at a time are sufficient to activate a group of muscles.

When the resistance or weight is increased gradually, your muscle will become stronger. However if you are looking to build large muscles rather than simply "tone" then you need to use some more extreme methods of isometric training which whilst being highly intense can deliver results which can rival those attained by people taking chemical steroids, especially if conducted whilst undergoing a planned supplementation regime using products such as Aminotaur which has been shown to naturally enhance muscle growth while you sleep.

Isometrics key advantage is that it can be performed without any specialised equipment. However if you want results faster and also you want to seriously increase your lean muscle mass then you can incorporate the basis of this with any strength training device ranging from chest expanders through to dumbbells and barbells. This type of training though is intense in nature if done correctly, therefore if you have high blood pressure or any sort of heart condition then consult your Doctor before training. If your doctor has any questions as this type of training is when done correctly can have numerous additional benefits, then tell him to contact us and we will gladly pass on any information that might help. Benefits of Isometric Exercises. Isometric exercises can be done without any kind of machines or equipment anytime, anywhere. If you have 10 seconds, you can work a muscle group without no one even noticing you are using isometric training. The convenience and time saving is one reason why isometrics are so popular and becoming even more popular as peoples lives get increasingly busy. Doing isometric exercises 7-10 seconds at a time during the day can substitute your workout -if done correctly. A bold claim? Yes it is but I feel confident in saying this. The simplest way to demonstrate this is by pressing your palms together as hard as you can, and holding the tension, will work your arms, shoulders and chest. To work your neck and upper back muscles, cross your fingers behind your head, push your head back in your hands using your neck muscles while trying to push your head forward with your hands. Find a wall to push up against or something you can pull against that won't move like a door jam. The only thing you need to remember is to use as much force as possible for 10 seconds. Using maximum force will give you all the benefits an isometric workout has to offer. Some proponents say to use 80% of your maximum - but how do you measure 80% and with my own studies I have never seen anyone hurt themselves using isometrics. If you have high blood pressure you should not engage in this type of activity because isometric exercises cause a spike in blood pressure. Although the blood pressure typically returns to normal rather quickly once the muscle is relaxed, the spike in blood pressure can be dangerous to those who already suffer from elevated blood pressure. If you suffer from high blood pressure but you really want to engage in isometric exercises, please consult with your doctor for tips on how to lower blood pressure first. Isometrics build muscle mass. In a recent experiment found an average size improvement of 12.4% for heavy isometric training and 5.3% with isometric training using weights equivalent to 60% of 1rm weight after a training period of 10 weeks. Using Isometrics For Strength To strengthen your bench press you could either get in a power rack and press the bar against an immoveable pin for a certain length of time, or hold a supra-maximal weight in a ¼ rep range for 6-20 seconds. The first type of isometric movement, pushing against an immoveable object, is used only for strength, whereas the 2nd type, holding a weight and preventing it from moving, is best for strength as well as muscle growth. Personally, I prefer the 2nd type where you simply hold a weight in place for both strength and muscle growth. Some say that when performing isometrics you will only strengthen the part of the movement you're training. For example if doing isometrics in a ¼ range bench press position you'll only strengthen that part of the movement. The truth is you will strengthen the part of the movement you're training, but you also get a 15-30 degree carryover and if you train at the most disadvantageous joint angle (like the bottom of a bench press or point in the squat where your thighs are parallel) you actually get a 100% strength carryover through the rest of the movement. Strengthen your weak links and everything else strengthens as well. In other words, if you perform an isometric contraction a few inches off your chest in the bench press you'll tend to increase the strength of your entire bench press and the size of your entire chest! But if you only do isometrics over the easiest ¼ or 1/3 range in a movement you only get a 15-30 degree carryover. If you really want to increase strength in a movement, using the bench press as an example, you'd simply use 3 different positions (bottom, mid-range, and top) and perform an isometric in each position. You'd perform isometrics in the contracted position near your chest, the midrange position, and then the extended position up top. A sample workout would be 2 sets of 10 seconds at each position with the lower position done first. For strength, each isometric contraction should last 20 seconds or less and ideally under 10 seconds. The benefits of isometric exercise are so many and varied yet simple and cheap to implement. Give them a go, you will notice improvements very quickly and can then make isometrics a key part of your exercise regime

The Benefits of Learning How to Build Muscle Without Weights

When was the last time you didn't cringe at the idea of doing another set of bench presses? Have you ever wondered if there is any such thing as gym equipment that is made for the average sized person? Chances are, having to deal with all kinds of complicated equipment is one of the main reasons why you stopped going to the gym. Fortunately, today there are training programs available to help you build muscle without weights. You should never deprive yourself of the kinds of exercise that will enable you to stay as strong and healthy as possible. That said, many people today erroneous believe that it is impossible to build muscle without weights. Oddly enough, humanity would be in a terrible predicament if bench presses and weight racks were part of daily existence. Without a question, if ancient humans needed to go to the gym, they would never have been able to hunt sabertooth tigers, let alone survive a whole host of other environmental factors. Across time, humans have found all kinds of natural methods for developing strong muscles, as well as keeping them. If it worked for them, why shouldn't it work for you? In order to learn more about how to build muscle without weights, you can start searching online. Chances are, you will find at least one program to work with. Are you ready to take back control of your physical fitness? Today, you don't have to sit around and look at a pile of exercise equipment that doesn't suit your needs. Why not try giving equipment free workouts a try? No matter how you look at it, you can't go wrong when you don't have to spend any extra money on products required for the regimen. Why let your body and your health go to rack and ruin? Muscle building and strength training can help just about anyone feel and look better. See my blog for more information, and then get clearance from your doctor.

FINAL WORDS

Always use proper form while exercising, remember - it's safety first. It is also recommended to stretch before and after your workout. Give these ideas a try, and never again have bully's kick sand in your face.

Good Training!

www.ingramcontent.com/pod-product-compliance
Lightning Source LLC
Chambersburg PA
CBHW061342120726
48001CB00002B/981